POUNDS LOSS
FOR THE JOURNEY

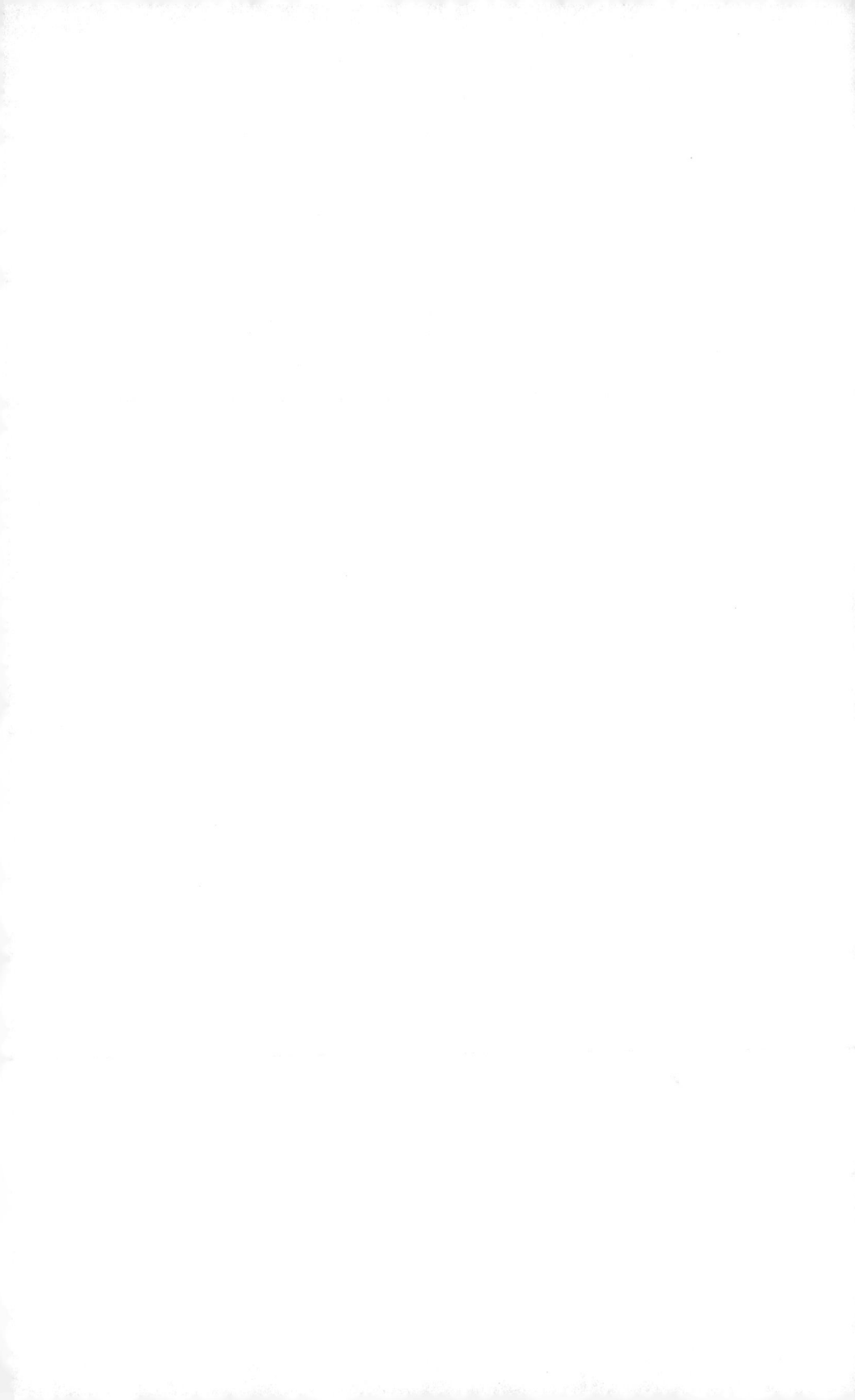

POUNDS LOSS FOR THE JOURNEY

God's Vision for Weight Loss

Pastor Jerrie Gillyard

Copyright © 2010 by Pastor Jerrie Gillyard.

Library of Congress Control Number:		2010900555
ISBN:	Hardcover	978-1-4500-2740-3
	Softcover	978-1-4500-2739-7
	Ebook	978-1-4500-2741-0

This book was printed in the United States of America.

To order additional copies of this book, contact:
Xlibris Corporation
1-888-795-4274
www.Xlibris.com
Orders@Xlibris.com
74052

ACKNOWLEDGEMENT

I want to give thanks to the following for being a blessing in my life. I thank God for His blessings. I praise God for being a keeper, a presence help and guiding me daily. There is none like Him.

To my prayer partners, you have always been there for me. Thanks for your faithful commmitment to God and to prayer. You are eternal treasures in my heart. The effectual fervent prayer of a righteous man availeth much. James 5: 16b.

To my brother and Sister-in-law, Deacon Robert and Gloria Gillyard, you have been a great inspiration.

To my niece, Cassandra, her husband (Minister Johnnie) and son (Joh'Shun) thanks for being my biggest supporter. Whenever I need you, you are always there. You are truly and inspiration.

I give thanks to my family, partners who have contributed to this ministry through words, love service, gifts, thoughts, encouragement, prayers and finance. It has been an uphill journey and I could not have made it without you.

To my niece, Tameka Martin and Husband, Carl and the three precious children, Tameka, you really blessed me, when you throught it all, went on to become a Register Nurse and a wonder wife and mother.

In loving memory of my father and mother Deacon Robert and Mrs. Estella Gillyard; who taught me that if you are going to do something in life, that will help others in a positive way, do it. and to my brother Jacob Gillyard who always was my shining light.

May God Bless and Keep You!

Pastor Jerrie Gillyard

CONTENTS

INTRODUCTION

A SHED WEIGHT loss journey you can afford is to help you lose the weight you desire, first I must tell you that it is not easily, but a willing mind and determine spirit must first be your focus and you must not be sidetrack to any circumstance that you will be facing in this journey of connecting with you mind and body.

Many have tried to lose weight and fail in their trying, my hope is that as you read this book it will help you to see yourself and be willing and determine to follow it and lose the weight you want. It was a struggle for me to meet the thirty days ahead but as I thought about the women's that would like to lose weight but fail in their trying, so I began to pray about what I could do to help and God lead me to start a connected journey and what type of food to eat and how to apply it so it would not be unhealthy for anyone.

The road to any journey is unknown until we start that journey and complete it. I knew that I would lose the weight because my mind and body was connected, when I took a hard seriously looks at myself in the mirror. It was as if I saw a bubble doll that has so many rolls of fat and at that time I only weighted one hundred and seventy-two, but as each day pass I was getting fatter and fatter. So I refused to let my body over rule my mind, it was a moment of tense and frustration, but then as I look and saw, I decide to do the impossible, and trust God for the possible.

It is a fact that no eating after 6:00pm or two hour before you retire to bed is because your metabolism slows down and what you eat and lie down will not burn of fat, and that morning will turn into fat, so you could not eat late at night while on this connecting journey. This is a sure way of knowing that you can shed some pounds off when you follow the menu as close as you can. All of this information is under girdle by the grace if God and my life experience and only what I did to accomplish this goal, I did not have a trainer, (could not afford one, even if I needing one) did not sign up for any program or exercise, did not go to the gym, but with the help of God All Mighty.

Now let me tell you about what I was around twenty-four seven, and that was food, because I served the seniors dinner five-days a week, did that cause me to forget my goal, no because I was determine to fight the temptation and with pray I was not tempted to eat. So the food did not get in my way to cause me to override what I started out to do. So if you are marry and have children that will not be a problem if you really want to lose pound. So go for it, feed your family what is necessary and eat as you are told in this book and your family will be so please, that you can take care of them and find time for yourself. So do what's important for you to bring more stability, and a more active, energize outgoing mother that bring balance to the family, and you will have more energy to do that you could not do before you lost the pound for the journey.

EXAMPLE: BALANCING MIND AND BODY

Let look at our checkbook, this is a reality for all of us that we have to face on a daily base. You have a balance of 2,000 dollar, and you went shopping and spent a sum of 900.00 dollar, you unmistaken forgot of the last week loan you made to your friend. Now you are about to balance your checkbook, everything is looking good and remember now the 150.00 dollar to the friend, your balance is 2,000 dollar, and you subtract the 900.00 dollar which left you a balance of 1,100 dollar, let's say the money is the mind and the balance is the body. Now you are to pay your house note which is 650.00, electric is 140.00 and your phone bill is 70.00, oh let's not forget the groceries bill which come to 130.00 so now you are ready to do a balance. You still need money for gas and others items but you are just reliant on your balance for that part.

But the main point of this example is to get you to see that the mind and the body must be in total balance and one cannot get ahead of the other. As I stated before the mind is the money and the body is the balance, let's dissect this for a minute: you see you were so intense on spending, like the mind is so yearning for more food, it want to eat, and the body is not in alignment with your mind so you do not notice it and guess what, you did not notice the increase of weight, the body is gaining and because the balance were not there . . . you, Whoop, gain some unwanted pound. So if you are to keep your focus on this journey to lose the amount of pound you want or just lose some weight you must stay balance in mind and body.

My Five-Month Experience: it's real and simple

April (thirty days, very important)

The thirty days is very crucial, because as you will learn in the book that this is where you train your body to become adjusted to the small portion, and certain type of food. And where most food is eliminated this transaction is taking place.

Five Months Grace Period

The five months Grace Period is not a time you can forget all about food for a while but only to open your list of food, and you will need God grace to help you to stay on course. Because now you can engage with more leafy vegetables and others side dishes in moderation and very small portion. Be very careful, the window is open. You will begin to feel better as you have accomplished your goal so far, but now yet. Stay encourages, pray that God will give you the strength and grace to stay focus.

May: the first month of the Grace Period
June: the second month of the Grace Period
July: the third month of the Grace Period
August: the fourth month of the Grace Period
September: the fifth and last month of the Grace Period

That's not the end, but now you can be open to choose on the food in the book and add other food that keeps you on the path to what you started out to do. Don't think that the five months is over and you can start eating whatever, because than you will defeat your purpose.

ABOUT THE AUTHOR

P ASTOR JERRIE GILLYARD-PITTS, a well-known inspirational motivator speaker and outgoing in her travel to reach a generation that is desperate for the one and only true God. She is the loving daughter of the late Mr. Robert Gillyard and the late Mrs. Estella Thomas Gillyard. Born in Mansfield, Louisiana where she grew up on a plantation and learn many tasks that she never through would be the pivot point of her most spectacular life today. After graduation, she moved to Shreveport, Louisiana where she went on to become one of the world highly professional cosmetology, after graduate from Helene Beauty School, and upon graduation she went on to become the owner of (2) beauty salon. During that time in 1979 she was called of God to preach the Gospel, some years later she enter St. Luke Missionary Baptist Bible College, where she received her Doctoral degree in theology. This truly was a turning point in her life, in 1980 when God spoke to her about white, gave her a vision with all color of clothes on a line, but among them all the white dress was more noticeable and what cause her to rise up and know that the white symbolize her call for her apparel now to dress in white, face with many obstacles that baffle her, infused her to go forth more boldly in her calling. Her call infused her to tackles some of the most critical problems and with God help she has stood the test of time. Her most concerned is the injustice of people on jobs that she is always confronted with, she never turned down a weary person who is facing a dilemma and her answer is always let's cry out to God. Many have been helped and she is willing to continue to help the misused, the rejected, the abused and the hurting. She went on to enter American School of Business to become a medical transcription, where she receives her diploma in the medical field.

She moved to Dallas, Texas in 1991, where she continues her work as a cosmetology, and work in the medical field as a file clerk. In her stay in Dallas, Texas she was called to preach in many churches and travels abroad. This was another turning point in her life, in 1997; she was led by the Holy Spirit to go back to her hometown Shreveport, Louisiana to start a ministry (On The Way Home Ministry), which would change her life. After four years in Shreveport, Louisiana she was led to Longview, Texas with the ministry and later back to Dallas, Texas. After eight years she moved to Denton, Texas where the ministry would become worldwide, she now has a television broadcast on Charter Cable and Verizon every Wednesday at 7:00pm and Sunday at 7:30pm. She host yearly women conference and fight for your health seminars. Her ministry "On the Way Home Ministries" reaching out to the homeless, nursing homes, hospitals and women shelters wherever the need is. The word of God was so clear as He spoke to her about encourage the people and to make sure they understand His word and how to apply it to their lives, because this generation is so far behind in the knowledge of His word. So as I wrote this book, my purpose is to open the eyes of many that they are not outcast but Godchildren or they can become His child as stated in Roman 10:9 said that if thou shall confess with thy mouth the Lord Jesus, and shall believe in thy heart that God hath raised Him from the dead, they shall be saved. God cares about all our problems and none is too big or small for Him to move on our behalf. Pastor Jerrie Gillyard-(Pitts) is single and has two sisters and two brothers.

FOREWORD

*   *   *

MINISTER JERRIE GILLYARD has always had a love for people and because her love for others she wanted to share what has worked to keep her healthy and lose unwanted weight.

In reading this book you will find the way to do this is to eat properly, moderation and spiritual commitment.

I congratulate her efforts and dedication to this project; she made sure the techniques she used worked for her before she shared it with others.

Marilyn Howard Freeman 2009

CHAPTER 1

The journey:
Obstacles along the way

I LIKEN THIS journey we all been waiting for, to the children of Israel: from so tired of trying to diet and lose weight and fail in trying, you can relax, no counting calories or choosing this or that food. This journey is somewhat similar to the journey of the children of the Israelites as they left the slavery of Egypt, please be aware there will be time of testing, but you will if you are determine and focus see the promise land. You know even in this life there are things we must face and go through to accomplish what God have for us, you see before God let the children of Israel go to the Promise Land that was flowing with milk and honey, God took them on a journey through the scotching desert of trials and testing. Deuteronomy 8:2-3 says, and you shall remember all the way which the Lord thy God led thee these forty years in the wilderness, to humble you, and to test thee, to know what was in thy heart, whether thou would keep his commandments, or not. 3. And he humbled thee, and suffered thee to hunger, and fed thee with manna, which thou knew not, neither did thy fathers know; that he might make thee know that man do not live by bread only, but by every word that proceed out of the mouth of the Lord doth man live.

In writing this book I was more concern as not to mention the word (DIET), because when we see diet, most of us refrain from it, due to the fact that we have or believe we have tried them all, or could I say done something in regard to dieting. But my emphasis is totally on eating small amount of food and certain type of food for thirty days and become adjusted to that style of eating and learn to withdrawn from your usually eating habit. For instance you have always has three meals a day whatever you wanting, you ate between meals, you ate much sweet during the day and there was no limit to the cold drink, and you I'm sure like myself, ate late at night. See just like the children of Israel, you will experience a deliverance from dieting and unnecessary food that may have has you bound for so long and kept you from coming to the promise land or reach your potential goal. This book is under girdle by God

Holy Spirit leading and my life experience as I obeyed His leading, and it will help millions to focus on their life in regard to their journey to shed weight loss. In this book you will learn how to follow in the footsteps of the children of Israel who arrived in the Promise Land of Milk and Honey.

Let's look at the Mighty Power of God, He deliverance the Israelites from the hand of Pharaoh, He parting the Red Sea, He provided a Lamb for Abraham, He spared the three Hebrew boys, God sent forth His only Son, that we may be free from sins. In John 8: 36 said, if the Son therefore shall make you free, ye are free indeed. Now you may not believe that God has anything to do with weight control but He does. If you turn to Him He will give you the desires of your heart, trust Him and let Him lead and direct you to your Promise Land. Your promise land is the place out of the desert where you used to be overcome with eating and has no control, but now that you have living truth and understanding how you can arrive to a place where you no longer feel temped to eat when you are not hungry. There will be time of testing alone the way, so remember the children of Israel, they were tested and fail at times, so prepare yourself for the trying time because there will be time when you see food and want to forget what you starting out to accomplish. See if your mind is made up and you believe in God, yes you can do this. I did it, not alone but with the help of God Almighty.

As you look at the children of Israel down in Egypt under such a hard taskmaster, they were in bondage for four hundred years and there only hope was for an answer that would help them to come out of what had them bound. And to them I'm sure they could do something only if there was someone who could reason with the uncontrollable Pharaoh. What I see about the children of Israel in their slavery in Egypt, is that what has them bound was what they only needing help to understand the cause, which was power from a devouring Pharaoh, which mean strength over time, because they has been there for so long, his power gave in to them and they believe that was there way of life.

It's the same problem we have with food; we are slaves to that power, which control us, and that is our eating habit. As it was with me, I was bound to my eating habit and only needing direction in what to do and how to do it. One day as I look at my clothes, which could no longer fix me, my mind was made up, girl do something-now. I knee and prayed to God for help, as I stood on Jeremiah 33:3 and cried out to God for encouragement and directions in what to. He led me by the function of the Holy Spirit to write this book. I pray that you find your promise land as you began your journey to shed some pounds.

CHAPTER 2

The Thirty Day Adjustment: Connecting the mind and body

REMEMBERING WHEN I was small in frame and healthier, I began to realize that the time is now to began my journey to losing weight and for health reason, also to lose so that I can help others to understand that it can be done without pills, counting calories, expenses diets, starvation, and over exertion of exercise, so my goal is to eat sensible and in moderation with some walking, which is good for health purpose, and drink plenty of water and rest. I began today 4/30/09 with this menu in mind. I really want to share exactly what I was led to do, so you can see that this in not just another book, but a way to guide you to a better way of life.

The Menu

My main menu for the first week only, of the thirty days
You can make adjustment to the food
For instance if you like cucumbers instead of avocados
Tomatoes
Red onions or white
Avocado
Plenty of Water
Tomato juice
Desert: Yoplait yogurt or cottage cheese with any fruit
Natural popcorn...................snack between meals
Small amount of grapes
Drink .... cinnamon tea

Side dish you can eat after one week in the pound loss journey: small portion
Boiled eggs
Cabbage-corns

Meats-fish, chicken, tuna salad
Green beans season
Broccoli/carrots
Green salad (small portion)
Bananas/peaches/crackers
Grapes (small amount)
Coffee with honey and cream (optional)

God gave us a choice, according to Roman 14:5 Let every man be fully persuaded in his own mind, we can decide for ourselves what is good and healthy for us so I began to use my mind to understand that I can do this, I began to believe I could lose weight if I make up my mind, so I did. Now the beginning was not easily but with the determination of connecting with mind and body it was a start. Once I dissected the meaning of the word determine, which mean to set your mind on a course of action. This kind of commitment means that you don't back out, but you work toward the goal you have set. If you have made a decision to follow the instructions in this book, don't allow excuses, distractions or second thoughts to deter you from your goal. I have struggle with weight problem for some time and I realize that if I did not do something I was on my way to disaster, but if you believe in the Bible like I do, you can do all things through Christ that strengthen you, knowing that God word is true the first step was not easily but the mind was made up. I had to look beyond and know that this is not just one day but many days were before me. Many opportunities to make choices will arise each day so I can be thoughtful and make choices that will lead to my greater wholeness. And with this in mind I was more determine.

The one thing I was determining to do was to rid fats out of this connected shed weight loss journey, as much as I could, but I could not do away with fat totally, because fat are used for many bodily functions and for the health of your hair. Yes, to much fat is bad for you: as you may or may not no that to many carrots at one time is not a good idea, because vitamin A is toxin in large quantities. So this journey will cause for some fat in moderation, this connected journey will allow you to enjoy all food categories, including fats and sweet in small portion if need be. After the thirty days and I suggest to give yourself another month which include the first five-months, before you bring in sweet. Unless you can do it in small portion, for instance: a slice of pie, eat only half of that. On this journey

I omit bread, drinks, coffee (one cup a day is reasonable), sugar, candies, potatoes, ice cream, cakes all types of chips and pies, only once a week you can eat a vegetables full balance meal, which includes meat. But you can eat two full meals a day if need be, only vegetables and fruits. After the first week I did not eat anything after 6:00pm or two hours before I retire to bed, because your metabolism slowed down when you are at rest and the food you eat will sure to turn to fat the next day. So be very careful of eating late at night.

First week: this is the test, to walk in the way God would have us, that mean we got to give up something, our worldly disposition, we must be willing to walk the straight and narrow path. It is the same with your health; there are some things you must give up to reach your goal, there are foods you will need to give up. In Matthew 16:24 Jesus said unto His disciples, if any man will come after me, let him deny himself, and take up his cross, and follow me. So we must understand this is not a (diet), it is that you are on a shed weight journey and you must be willing to give up that which is harmful to you. This may cause you to fail. A thought: (your life is what you make of it, if it don't fix; you need to make alteration). This is what need to be done on the connected journey, is to make alteration in your eating habit.

First day: well it's on now; woke up feeling very strong, has no breakfast, went for a forty-five minute walk, came back, and went out window shopping and walk outside for about four hour and came back home late that evening and prepared my first meal, drink plenty of water, and snack. After 6:00pm I developed a headache, but that was because my body was adjusted the change of food and eating habit, I did not take anything for it; I retired for the night, and that morning no headache.

Second day: no headache, did not walk, I ate one Yoplait yogurt, drink plenty of water and I went to Church, praise God for all that He has done for me. Return home and ate my usually meal, feeling good; did not walk but did a few house shores and about 4:00pm I has my snack and plenty of water and some cinnamon tea drink, feeling real good.

Third day: woke up feeling a little weak, ate Yoplait yogurt and went for a forty-five minute walk, came back, resting for a while and drink plenty of water. I did some studying and computer work. And I began to prepare my meal; I also did some house shores. The hungry pangs began about 10:00am; I began to get a little weak so I eat my meal. After the meal I began to feel a little at ease and my hungry pangs went away. It seems that my strength was building up, I drink plenty of water, and I felt very strong in my and body.

In this connected journey I learn that you must keep busy or your mind will lead you to do something other than consecrate on what you have deciding to do. Your body in other word will react to feeling tired, weary, and weak; you will begin to crave for other food. When mind and body react differently that is an unbalance situation, you must keep focus on your goal and keep active in body. When the two began to go their separate way that when I get my Bible and study, or go walking and believe me it work. It brings my mind and body together; there is the connected link. The mind must always be in dominion of the body to bring it in line with your thinking. You will need to be encouraged as you focus, this was my lead that really encourages me, I will accept an opportunity today to act as if I can handle a situation I used to run from.

We must learn to do all things in moderation as the Bible tells us in Philippians 4:5, which said let your moderation (being satisfied with less than one's due) be known unto all men (even our enemies). The Lord is at hand (is near; actually refer to the rapture) which include our eating habits. The point is to keep busy and focus on what your goal is. And I believe that you can make it with prayers. Just remember success is when the mind (heart) changes, and then the body will follow.

Fourth day: woke up this morning refresh and strengthen, has prayer, ate one Yoplait yogurt and went for a forty-five minute walk and return home and did many house shores that needed to be done. Drink plenty of water kept very busy and at noon ate my usually meal and drink cinnamon tea. Did more work on the computer, rested for a while. That night I was feeling so wonderful and good in spirit, mind and body I went to bed and slept so well, thank God for all His help and Holy Spirit that enable me to keep focus on my heart desire.

Fifth day: oh it is so wonderful, after a good night sleep woke up feeling like I was on a road to somewhere, but not knowing where but in my spirit I knew it was God Holy Spirit leading me to my destiny where I really desire to be, and that is stay on focus to lose weight, although I cannot see pounds shedding of but in my mind I knew it was going to happen. Took a forty-five minute walk came back, ate one Yoplait yogurt, feeling very good, prayed and thank God Almighty for his blessings and began study. I went to get some vegetables I needing for my usually meal. No headaches just feeling great on my weight loss journey.

I ate my usually meal at 12noon, and was still ready to go, because I felt so good and strong in my mind and body so I began to study God word and meditate on what I study. For dinner I has a small portion of corn and baby carrots. Went for a thirty-minute walk before retiring to bed I has snack, (small portion of popcorn) slept good that morning I began to pray and thank God for His strength that lead me day by day.

Sixth day: whooping, I feel so wonderful and strong in mind and body, when I got up this morning I said thank you God, and prayed. Was still for a while then I ate one Yoplait yogurt and did some work on my computer, be sure stay active. Study God word and concentrate on what I have study. Mind so stay on what I have been leads to do and that is stay connected to my goal to lose weight.

Seven day: feeling a little tired, weak and hungry but I knew it will be this way until I get more time into this journey, so I went right on and did house shores and did not go walking, so I ate one Yoplait yogurt and went out for a drive and back home.

Began to meditate on the word of God and has prayer, and I felt much better. At night is when I really have no appetite at all, and I will eat a small portion of popcorn or Yoplait yogurt and about two hour after I will retire to bed. This is the first week of the shed pound journey, I did not deter or binge in anyway because I am determine to help others to do that which many have tried but fail due to lack of understanding and knowledge.

Second week: this is the flip side of the shed weight loss journey, this is when your mind must be anchor and firm in this change, because this is the time you maybe led to over indulge, but don't because this is the time you can introduce other foods in your journey, but in moderation only. A thought: God want us to learn how to rise above the magnetic pull of the refrigerator so that food does not consume our lives. What made me want to keep going on this weight loss journey was that you have that time of choosing different foods and not just eating the same food all the time.

Success is when the mind (heart) changes, and then the body will follow. You are a success when you changed your mind attitude toward food, and it is starting to affect the way you eat. You are a success because of the behavior changes, the one thing I learn in this connected journey is that after the first week you will be more less apt to eat as you were during that first week, so just stay on course and put God first and yes you can do it. This second week for me was a blast because I did not want to eat anything else, but what I ate in the beginning. It may not be this way for you, but remember to stay on focus.

Eight day: this is the second week into my shed weight journey, this is where motivation began here, because you are so over the yearning and need for food that you are now ready for the journey, that all you have on your mind is to stay on course for the complete journey. Your body is now adjust to the usually of what you now are eating. This morning I was feeling real good, went out walking came back and ate one banana and one Yoplait yogurt. I now am ready to do some Bible studying.

Ninth day: has a night of restless due to the vitamin C that I began to take for building up my immune system, at the time I did not know that due to he change in my eating habit was the cause of the effect. But after that morning I was all right, I continue to take the vitamin C and it really boost my strength. I ate one boil egg and drink plenty of water, and ate lunch my usually meal and felt very well. But I do have a true story to tell because I was traveling and needing some water, so I tested myself and stop at a chicken place, oh I tell you the smell of that chicken was astounding and I kept focus only got water and back on the road, when I arrive home I was so over whelm about my reaction. I thank God for his strength that help me to overcome the temptation. I was a little hungry so I ate one bananas and one peach and retired to bed after two hour.

Tenth day: woke up feeling good, ate two boil eggs and off for walk about forty-five minute, came back and did work in office and some house shores. I was feeling well and vigor so I decide to relax for a while. Now my mind is more on studying the word of God and food is not my first choice. In my mind I know now that some weight has shed and in my body, I can feel light and not puffy, if you know what mean. Because like me if you are fat, or over weight, no matter what you put on you feel big and stuff. But since I started this shed weight loss journey I feel so much better in mind and body, the fact is I even look better.

Eleventh day: blessed morning, as all God's days is, feeling real good and ready for the day a little weak in body as the morning progressed. But drink water and ate my first meal an hour before noon, collar green and for desert one peach. Did not walk today did much house shores and study for some time. There are times when you will began to feel hungry, but remember that is natural, because you are not eating the way you used to. So if you began to get hungry, eat some fruit or Yoplait yogurt, always keep it on hand as an emergency helper. When hungry pangs came what I did (concerning food) was eat one fruit and plenty of water, which help to flush your system out, and believe me that really cause you to feel good.

Twelfth day: woke up, had prayer, went for a walk about forty-five minute, and I felt so successfully because I run for a while and came back home, ate usually meal for lunch and drink water, cinnamon tea and relax by study my Bible. Did some housework and then got on the computer for ministry work. This really has been as all others days very blessed and I really thank God for the strength and encouragement for this journey.

Thirteen day: wow! It is wonderful and I am praising God for His goodness and mercy. Well I went for a forty-five minute walk and did some running not much but just to stay in practice. I return home and ate one peach and at noon my usually meal, and drink plenty of water. Then I relax and began study and did some house shores. It was very exciting because

Fourteen day: up and prayed, I ate one banana drink plenty of water. Went out walking and looking, came home ate popcorn and got on computer. Study

God word and starting to work on computer and did some house shores. This is the last day that I will need to eat very strictly because after fourteen days you can assimilate others food on the menu into your weight loss. I can say it has not been easy but thank to our Heavenly Father He has been with me from the beginning and gave me the strength that I needing to go forth. There were time I thought I could not make it, but with the determination and willingness I kept my focus and stayed on course. See your thirty days is the main focus, because it will lead you to stabilize and adjust your body for the five-months ahead.

Third week: the third week in your connected weight loss is now wise spread, because you can eat others food on the menu, such as steak, green (any kind), pinto bean (any kind), pimento cheese, rice, tomato juice, sometime I would only drink a glass for lunch), be sure if you need a balance breakfast, you can in moderation. Don't forget that you have not completed your thirty-days, and you must keep focus, you are not ready to indulge in other food yet, but what on the thirty-day menu.

Fifteen day: well this was like a new start again but I held my posture and remember the connection, I went walking for forty-five minute and run some which I can say an hour of exercise. Did usually housework and computer, with mind on how far I have come; it really made me feel good about this whole ordeal. I ate the usually and drink plenty of water. That afternoon I had some steak and vegetables with lots of water. For snack I have plain popcorn, I was feeling very strong and vigorous from the change of food that I has been eating but it was good.

Sixteen day: today is amazing, whoopee, I ate one peach and off for a walk, as I walk I began to think of how this weight loss came to me and it was through prayer that led me to have faith in God and start with the process. Return home ate lunch that including steak, corn and water. Studying for a while and relax than I has a snack which was plain popcorn and water. I went for a late evening walk and return home and relax. Did some computer work. For dinner I ate usually meal. Were feeling good and my body adjusted well with the change of food?

Seventeen day: all is well, very happy and ready to continue because it is fantastic.

PASTOR JERRIE GILLYARD

This is so good that I really have no desire for any sweet, drinks and it really is good to know that you can succeed in what you have a mind to do to help others along the way. I now only crave what my usually menu call for and guess what, it is not expenses and you can afford it.

Eighteen day: today I was feeling weak, but I went for a walk for about forty-five minute and return home, ate some crackers, pimento cheese, drink plenty of water. About noon I prepared my usually meal, tomatoes, and avocados and drink plenty of water. I did house shores and computer work. One thing I need to mention is that you must keep busy doing active work, walking, shopping and visiting but above all you can pray and study God word. Because when I began to feel hungry, besides eating I get the Bible and study, about thirty minute you do not want anything to eat. If our minds are focus on what we are doing, that urge will go away, believe me I have has to face that problem many time.

Ninth-teen day: thinking about the time has come for me to do a big turn over in this connected shed weight loss my mind was shouting and my body wanting to run. I arise refresh and went for a walk and run for about forty-five minute. Return and ate crackers and pimento cheese drink plenty of water. Relax and got busy doing housework and computer work, the day was extremely wonderful and I ate my meal at 11:00pm, the menu was: corn and bake chicken small portion.

Twentieth day: another wonderful time in my life as I am more interested in what the result will be. At this time I am thinking a scale and shouting because I know that my faithfulness and hard work will not be in vain. But I could not be thinking about this right now, but yes it is on my mind. But I began to consecrate to bring a balance by remembering that mind and body is the main object here.

Twenty-one day: this is coming to the end of my third week on this connected journey and I am more happy and ready to continue on through, because it now has been almost a month. For breakfast I ate crackers and cheese. For lunch my usually avocado, tomatoes and plenty of water, cinnamon tea. Went for a walk that afternoon, and was so full of energy. My time is now more on praying and study God word. A thought: some time its worst to win a fight than to lose.

Fourth week: as the journey continues, I am more anxious to engage in it more faithful and be very careful of what I eat. I will stay with the complete food items that was including in this shed weight-loss journey. As I came to the fourth week it was more pressure so you got to watch it, because you may want to binge, but I hope you are focus as I was, you could be more careful and stay with the menu. You cannot eat more because this is the last week, you must remember the journey is not over, there are five more month ahead, not as leaning as the thirty-day was, but you can't eat what you want at this moment in the journey, and it is a good way to indulge but this is the critical moment, so stay on course.

Twenty-two day: this day I have the opportunity to make out my list of what I will eat for this last week and two days, oh! Was I excited and was even more willing to keep my focus, because I have come this far and for sure I will not cop out now. For breakfast I has one Yoplait yogurt. My meal for today was bake chicken and crackers, plenty of water. My body was feeling very good about 5:00pm I ate popcorn for snack.

CHAPTER 3

Prayer and Studying God word was my first priority

THERE IS NO doubt that it is by praying that we learn to pray, and that the more we pray, the better our prayers will be. People who pray in spurts are never likely to attain to the kind of prayer described in the Scriptures as "powerful and effective" (James 5:16).

Great power in prayer is within our reach, but we must work to obtain it. We should never even imagine that Abraham could have interceded so successfully for Sodom if he had not communed with God throughout the previous years of his life.

So before I began to step out, I remember to pray and ask God to direct me in the way that He would have me to go. As He direct I follow and was obedient to His voice.

If you are discouraged I have news for you—good news. You do not need to continue so, not at all. There is a way to end discouragement. And the word itself gives the clue.

Putting the prefix dis before the word courage forms "Discouragement",

Which mean a discounting of courage? Therefore the way to end discouragement is to remove the prefix and to lay under your life a solid foundation of courage. Winston Churchill, that marvelous genius in the use of the English language, expresses it well. He says, "Success is never final. Failure is never fatal. Its courage that counts, so instead of counting calories, you must count on your courage to pray and reach your goal in losing your weight desire.

The Prayer Of Faith

How are we to ask? Jesus says: therefore I tell you, whatever you ask in prayer, believe that you have received it, and it will be yours (Mark 11:24). You not only speak to the problem of your weight, believing it will shed.

You also speak to God, believing that you have received what you ask. And Jesus says: "it will be yours." You speak to the God of promise, who always keeps His word.

'Whatever' here, literally means, 'all thing,' including your weight problems. All the things that you ask God in prayer to give you will be yours. When you ask, you are to believe that you have already received the answer to your prayer. You can only believe like that, if you know that God wants to give you that particular thing for which you ask, if the spirit witnesses that truth to your heart. You will not find it easy to believe that you have already received it unless you know the utter faithfulness of God in keeping all the words of the covenant that He has established with His children.

CHAPTER 4

How to Create a More Peaceful, Simpler Life from the Inside Out

L ET'S LOOK AT the story of Daniel, and this will help you to know that without God you can do nothing of yourself but all is possible with God. Now this story is not to change your mind or lead you as Daniel did, but to encourage you that when God is in the midst nothing is impossible. In chapter one of Daniel in that twelfth verse through the twenty verses read as follows: 12. Prove you servants, I beseech you, ten days; and let them give us pulse (vegetables) to eat, and water to drink. You see Daniel proposed a test of "ten days" during which they would be given only vegetables to eat and water to drink. This didn't mean that Daniel and the others were vegetarians, but rather that the meat provided by the Babylonians was unlawful to eat because of being unclean, or else it was not properly prepared!) 13. Then let our countenances be looked upon before you, and the countenance of the children who eat of the portion of the king's meat: and as you see, deal with your servants. 14. So he consented to them in this matter, and proved them ten days. (Evidently) the Lord told Daniel to do this. The Lord also helped Daniel, because otherwise ten days would not be enough time to show much either way.) 15. And at the end of ten days their countenances appeared fairer and better in flesh than all the children, which did eat the portion of the king's meat. 16. Thus Meltzer took away the portion of their meat, and the wine that they should drink; and gave them pulse, which mean vegetables. (It is evident that the Lord took a hand in the proceedings.) 17. As for these four children, God gave them knowledge and skill in all learning and wisdom, and Daniel had understanding in all visions and dreams. ("God gave," refers to the proclamation by the Holy Spirit that the three years of their training in all the sciences and arts of Babylonian learning did them no good whatsoever. It was the Lord who gave them what they needed.) 18. Now at the end of the days that the king had said he should bring them in, then the prince of the eunuchs brought them in before Nebuchadnezzar. (When these young men stood before Nebuchadnezzar, the ruler of the world, little did the Monarch realize how prominently four of them, and especially Daniel, would figure in the remainder of his life.) 19. And the king communed with them; and among them all was found none like Daniel, Hannah, Michael, and Azariah: therefore stood they before the king. (The king found "these four children" were far superior to all others). 20. And in all matters of wisdom and understanding, which the king enquired of them, he found them ten times better than all the magicians an astrologers who were in his entire realm. (This is astounding considering that these four were still only boys, probably still in their teen years or in their early twenties at the most.)

This will help as you look at Daniel life and others that were with him, how they ate only vegetables and water. So as God by the Holy Spirit directed me in this plan of eating for thirty day, is not surprising to me, because he is the same Lord now as He was then. The Bible tells us in Hebrew 13:8 He is the same God today, yesterday and forever. And this is not as fast as some may think, but this is a way to help many to lose weight in a normal and natural way. The only different in Daniel and us is that you can include many others foods then vegetables and water, much more to add to our countenance and health as well. Despite our best effort to do that, which is right, we at least can be aware of the pitfalls that lied ahead. So on this journey just know that there will be days that you may binges some, but remember to keep focus, pray, studied God word.

I know ten days is not a long time, but just imagine Daniel and his friends only eating vegetables and water, but we have a variety of vegetables, fruits, meat, and others food. The countenance of our appearance may not change, but we will shed some pound on the outside and our inside will be natural healthy, and we can say thanks to God for instructed someone who has a heart to consider others in a plan of natural means to lose or shed some pound

Twenty-three day: well this is the last week of my journey and do you know it is a blessing in disguise. I am so thankful and ready to see what the end will be, but guess what? It's not over just because you are done with the thirty days, but you must watch what you eat and not forget that the journey is not over until you are at your desire weight loss. The journey was to train your mind and body that you can and you will. So keep focus and eat sensible and yes you now can add more vegetables, fruits, if you like but stay on course. You have come this far; don't blow it now. Many time the only way I persevered was prayer and been reminded that I made it thus far I can't stop now, and that what kept me going.

Twenty-four day: today it is raining and I am up and really for the day, I prayed and thank God for His blessings. My breakfast was two Yoplait yogurts and water; I was feeling good and wonderful. I studying for a while and then I began to read over my manuscript and correct, edit and add to the writing. My lunch was: pinto beans, rice and baked chicken, drink plenty of water. Oh! I felt good.

Twenty-fifth day: what a blessing it is to be almost to the end of my thirty-day journey to lose some pound. It really has been fun and exciting to learn that whatever you set your mind to do, you can. I am so excited and feeling like I have did something that I have never done before, but I have dieting many time and for long period of time, but never consider the natural way and connected mind and body to this extinct. I have not ever ate like this and it really been good just knowing that when you are seriously about wanting to lose some pounds you can pray and ask God for His leading, and study His word for guidance and you will be overwhelm with what the outcome will be. Just keep your focus on the main goal, you are not dieting, but you are eating less and natural and determine to shed weight and feel good on the inside and pound loss on the outside for your overall health.

Twenty-six day: the time is right, why because I feel good and everything is been held together, and this morning I went for a forty-minute walk, it was a beautiful day, misty a little and walking in the mist was good. I ate one Yoplait yogurt for breakfast, drink plenty of water, and went out visiting and back home. I did some house work and computer work. You know since this shed weight-loss journey began, and my changed of eating, now I don't even think about other food. It not a need there anymore and I am so happy because I can do whatever I put my mind to do and with the help of God you can make it to.

Twenty-seven day: went for a forty-five minute walk, came back and relax has no breakfast, was not hungry, so I study and prepare for an outing. Came home got on computer, this day was very exciting to me because I did not want anything to eat. But at dinner I had a complete salad and drink plenty of water. Now I know why I am not hungry, because I am almost to the end of the thirty days.

Twenty-eight day: well the thirty day journey is about over and I am a happy person, all because I can't believe that I really did keep my focus. Thank God for His hand of mercy that was with me all the way. This morning I ate no breakfast, just to exciting I guess, but drink plenty of water, don't forget the water. At dinner I has a complete salad, (did not include meat), and water.

Twenty-ninth day: hallelujah! This is the day I been waited on, because one more day and I can say when your mind and body is in alignment you can do whatever your heart desire with the help of God who will lead and direct you to your destiny. God is so good and merciful unto us. This morning I went for an hour walk, I feel so good in mind and body that I am walking more now than before, thanks to God for He made it all possible for me and He can do it for you. Luke chapter 1:37 said, for with God nothing shall be impossible. I did not want anything to eat after my walk, I began to studying and pray that God strength will hold me for the next five month, and I believe with all my heart, soul and mind that He will, He never fail.

Thirty day: breakfast: one boiled egg, plenty of water, lunch: baked chicken with rice and peas. And I began to think of the journey of weight loss I was more determining to hold fast to my decision. I went for an evening walk for forty-five minute. For snack plain popcorn and plenty of water.

This is the last day of the thirty days, so I am very happy and blessed because I could not have done it alone, thanks to God Almighty for been there for me. Prayed and study more that I would be able to continue the shed weight-loss journey. Because there are five months ahead, and I do not want to be led in any way that will affect the rest of the journey. My weight was at the beginning one hundred and seventy-two pound, but as of today my weight now register at one hundred and sixty-five pound, hallelujah, thank God for the strength and faith that He provided for me. I lost seven pounds in thirty day, with the menu that if you are willing and determine you can do the same. The goal is to stay focus on the first thirty-day menu and only the foods that are in this book for the shed weight-loss journey.

CHAPTER 5

The Five-Month Journey

THE FIVE-MONTH IS when you must consider that, you made it thus far and are willing to continue for the ultimate result. Now the first of the five-month, I must warn you, that you be very careful in following the food in this book, you will have a variety of food to choose from. So don't think the journey is over, because really this is the extreme testing time, keeping in mind the children of Israel in the wilderness. My first month which for me was May 1 to May 30, so I began my first month with Yoplait yogurt, tuna salad, crackers, grits, butter and sausages, small amount of cheese, until about the third week is when I adding others food on the menu in this book. I would prepare a well balance meal once a week; you can do two if you need to, but my well balance meal including food such as: rice, bean, chicken or ground chunk and plenty of water. Just remember each month cause you to add others food, but not if it is not listed in the book. It was in the last week of my first month that I began to drink natural Snapple, with one meal a day. I also included tuna salad with crackers and I began to drink one cup of coffee in the morning with honey and cream. Now the second month of the five-month journey, I was hesitating to bring in sweet, because the calories would overrule my plan for now. The honey in the coffee is ok, because honey in itself was noticeable in recent years, but has taken a back seat to man-made antibiotics and to processed sweeteners. But modern science shows honey kills bacteria that even the most powerful antibiotics can't handle. And since it contains traces of vitamins, minerals, proteins, and others nutrients—which sugar don't have—it is the sweetener of choice again for many people. My weight now is one hundred and sixty two, and this is only my second month of the five-month.

Into the third month, I call this the high rising journey because you are now coming up the mountain and slowly adding other food to the shed weight loss journey. You are regaining your strength and your body is now adjusted to the small amount of food, and due to the change in the first two-month you are well able to sustain your craving for food you don't need. Remember you can eat snacks listed in this book when you feel a cause to do so. Now the third month you can add cheese, crackers, salmon and tuna salad, cottage cheese with fruits. And for midnight snacks you can have small portion of raisins. Always remember you still must remain the small portion. Let say you are in the third month, your breakfast if need be could be: Yoplait yogurt, or two boiled egg, or small amount of grits with butter and sausages.

And your lunch (optional) could be baked chicken or fried, turkey or fish (one piece) rice and fresh peas or can peas, green (any kind) and for desert, sliced peaches. Maybe you need a late snack: natural popcorn, or raisins, one fruit, two hours before you retire for the night. March, the month I usually cook chicken dressing, I knew this would be a problem, but it was not because I remember the goal I starting and yes I has a wonderful meal which was, turkey dressing (my first time to eat bread since I starting the Pound Loss for the journey), cranberry sauce, green beans and for dessert (bananas pudding). And plenty of water was my drink.

The fourth month, what do you to now, well it a pleasure because you can look on the menu in this book and choose your choice, that's a blessing. Maybe now you are craving some sweets, we'll try some beets, because they have the highest sugar content of any vegetable. In fact, 40 percent of the world's refined sugar come from beets. Unlike sugary desserts, this brightly colored root is low in calories and high in nutrients. Beets are loaded with potassium, magnesium, beta-carotene, and foliate, one of the B-vitamins. These nutrients can help keep your heart healthy and your bones strong. They can even prevent cancer.

The fifth month, first let's praise God for this pounds loss for the journey, this is not he end, but you are coming to the close of your last of the five month, what a blessing this has been. Now you can assimilate all foods listed in this book, what you would like to eat, but remember you must stay focus on you goal of pounds loss for the journey, it not over yet, consider your weight and how much you want to loss. Walk as much as you can alone the way for it will keep your mind clear and your body in tone. Your menu must be simple and in small portion until you know that you have reached your promise land, and that is your desired pounds loss. My weight now is one hundred and fifty, WHICH WAS MY GOAL: PRAISE GOD.

Simple menu for the five-months

Baked chicken	Tuna salad	Fish: baked or fried	Cottage cheese
Rice	Crackers	Corn	Peaches, raisins
Green peas	Snapple drinks	Broccoli	Orange juice
Sliced peaches	Steak	Yoplait yogurt	Popcorn

Remember you must stay away from potatoes, any type of chips, bread, cakes, candies, cookies, ice cream soft drinks and others food you know that are not recommended in this book. You want to reach your desired weight, so do not over indulge in what's not in the book. These are example of food I ate and you may create your own, but stay focus, you have come this far while not finish with pounds loss for your journey. Let me ask you a question, what will you do now that the five-month is complete? Will you say, I have lost the pounds, now I can eat whatever I want to, or will you say, now the pounds is off, I can eat ice cream and drink cold drink as often as I want to, or now I thank God for His help and I will be obedience and not indulge in what I know will cause me to do as Israel did after they left slavery. THINK ABOUT IT.

CHAPTER 6

Why the five Months
The Grace of God

I N ISAIAH 40:31 but they that wait upon the Lord shall renew their strength; they shall mount up with wings as eagles; they shall run, and not be weary; and they shall walk, and not faint. This is where Grace begin, why: because the number five mean (God Grace) and according to Ephesians 2:5 said, even when we were dead in sins, hath quickened us together with Christ, (by grace you are saved). So since we are save by God grace, and grace is God unmerited love toward us, I believe it will take God grace to help you through, God Grace help me through this pound loss for the journey. In 2 Corinthians 9:8 And God is able to make all Grace abound toward you (presents the ability of God); that you, always having all sufficiency in all things (mental, physical, economical, and spiritual), may abound to every good work (using God's blessings for the good of others).

During the first month after the thirty days of your journey you need not be discourage because grace will see you through. We know in life there is such a thing as an upbeat and a downbeat, Psalms 42:5 Why are thou cast down, O my soul? And why are thou disquieted in me? Hope thou in God: for I shall yet praise him for the help of his countenance. Life is what we make of it; if it doesn't fix you make alteration. You may not have lost the weight you wanted even at three months, there is still time and the five months is where you can make alterations. That mean you may have to alienate some food or you may need to add more, whatever you do, don't let discouragement stop you, this is normal, each month you can add others food to your menu. For instance for the first month you may add some of the thirty-day menu. But granting the fact of mood, we as individuals are not relieved from the responsibility of maintaining power over discouragement.

In the Bible in the book of 3 John 2 tell us, Beloved, I wish above all things that you may prosper and be in health, even as you soul prospered. That while I prayed and ask God to guide me so that this book will be a source of strength to all and it will help you to become the person you so desire just by following the menu and eating what already in your house or that is costly for you. The food is what you make of it, what I mean is you really can eat what you have a taste for in moderation and using your mind and body to dictate to you that this is enough and don't forget to stay focus on what your purpose is, and that is to lose the pounds for the journey. Let your journey be successful. Mine was . . .

PASTOR JERRIE GILLYARD

CHAPTER 7

My Five-Month Journey

MY FIRST MONTH: may 1-31, so well please at the result of the thirty-days Pound loss journey, I lost eight-pounds. The first month was easy because my body is well adjusted to less food. There was no craving or wantonness; I began with a very small portion of eating others food now introduces into the first month. I am very optimistic about what I eat and how much, well my first month include meat, (only chicken and ground chuck), vegetables, fruits, beans, green, rice, broccoli, you can always include any food on the thirty-day menu at anytime. Your first month if you like can have cold drinks, only once a month or I prefer, Snapple drink which you can have every other day. You can eat one, two or three meals a day. Very small portion will keep you on course. I will haste to say, yes you can eat out just remember your desire and be modest about choosing your menu.

My choice was for each weeks, I would eat one or two small portion meal for four days and for three day I would eat three small meals, for example: breakfast, one boil egg, coffee with honey and cream, and crackers. Lunch, I desire a light meal due to my body was so well stable that I only needed a very small portion of foods like: one chicken leg, or ground chuck, with rice and vegetable (your choice). Dessert: Yoplait yogurt and for snack I would eat a bag of popcorn. Before six o'clock I would eat other small meals for dinner.

Please don't forget to drink plenty of water. And remember not to eat late at night. I always prayed and ask God our Heavenly Father, to help me to stay on course and He did and will do the same for you. So just stay focus and keep your mind and body balance because the pounds loss for the journey is still on until you like myself, reach your promise land of slim and trim.

The second month June 1-30, I was very pleased because I could add other food from the menu or perhaps include some other vegetable or fruit. As long as you stay within the limit of foods that you can eat, as not to indulge in food that are not appropriate for your journey. For instance like ice cream or cakes (small amount if need be). Most of the second month I ate for breakfast: eight crackers, four slices of cheese and one cup of decaffeinated coffee. For lunch I would eat cottage cheese and peaches or pineapples or strawberries. Some days I would eat a balance meal like: if not cottage cheese it would be for Lunch: baked chicken or steak with rice and beans, or your choice of vegetables. The third month: July 1-31, you can include some roast peanut and orange juice in small portion. Adding others food to your menu is guiding by how much weight you have lost or how much you would like to lose. The fourth month: August 1-30, is where you can still add others food in this book to your menu. I consider eating more fruits and vegetables, because since my body is now well adjusted to eating small portion, which made it possible for the weight to come off.

The fourth month August 1-30, oh how I really enjoyed the timing of waiting for this month, I can relax and concentrate on all that I in the strength of the Lord Jesus who help me to stay on course as I progress through this pound loss for the journey. I began to open up and add others food in the menu in this book and what a blessing it was for me, and it will be for you to. I began to cook more and stayed in the limit of foods that I could eat. Sometime I would cook a full balance meal that include, beans, rice, steak smothered and drink one Snapple.

You can now realize how much or less food you can intake now, because you can see the result. Let me pause to say, it depend on your weight and how much you desire to lose, you're eating habit may not be as mine, you will have to consider that, and do the alteration in subtraction or adding how much you can intake.

Your Promise Land
Hallelujah! I've Lost ____ Pound on my Journey

Now the time is winding down, don't blow it now, your journey is not over but coming to an end. This month, which is the fifth month: September 1-30, is time now to be careful of not losing the way, because it set the tone for your outlook on your life, health and weight. You must exercise your mind and body not to aviate from the menu in this book; you can add other food to your meal, but only what listed in the book. I did not forget what was important to my success in losing weight. Extra-ordinary! You bet, your journey was the hand of God that got you through to your promise land as where you can eat in moderation and because your body is so well adjust to eating certain and small portion of food. You know many time I would fill my plate with all kinds of food and guess what? I would only take two spoon of each vegetable and four bite of meat and truly did not want any more, I have come to that point now that food is not what will hold me in bondage, but now I know that I can control what is before me and that is because of my mind and body have so well been effected by the thirty-day connective journey and now I can and hope that you can give all thanks to God for impressing a concern and caring woman who herself experience this magnificent journey to help those in need of living to eat healthy and lose the pound. Tell someone else about your victory in Pound Loss for the Journey. The Bible said, when you are blessed, we could bless others, SO THIS IS MY GIFT TO YOU.

CHAPTER 8

Food you have a choice to select and what you must avoid:

For the first month (thirty-day) menu only

Tomatoes
Avocados
All vegetables (small portion)
All fruits (2 a day or mix with cottage cheese)
Raisins (one half cup or less)
Grapes (small amount)
Cottage cheese
Yoplait yogurt
Cinnamon tea (one cup a day)
(Receipt for tea: cinnamon stick, boil until ready, strain.
You can drink hot or cold. Refrigerate).
Tomato juice 1 8oz glass
Plenty of water

YOU MUST AVOID: for the first month, if possible the food that have a star, you must not eat during the first month. Try to avoid if possible throughout the journey, it will help you to lose weight more rapidly.

Potatoes* (A must)
Ice cream*
Bread* (A must)
Candies*
Cold drinks*
Alcohol*
Chips
Pies*
Cakes*

Cheese (small portion)
Grapes (can be eat throughout the five-month)

I N ALL FAVOR do not deter from the following list of food, because this is what helped me to lose my desire weight. You can if you desire to choose others food beside what is listed, but be sure that if you refused grapes, get cherries or plums. Just be sure to remain as closed to the menu and food items listed in this book.

In your third week of the first month in the journey, you can begin to add small portion of meats, and crackers and cheese.

Fourth week you must stay connected to the usually meal that you begin with, because you will be tempted to eat more, but it not the time to indulge now you must keep focus and be moderate in what you eat so that the THIRTY DAYS be equal to your starting day in the shed weight loss journey and believe God for the strength that you need. Remember that you will or may not be feeling good in body, when you first began to eat or add more certain food to the menu, your body may take a turn to adjust to the increase of food, but it is natural.

After the first month of the shed weight loss journey, you cannot rush into eating whatever you want to. There is still time for that; you are still in training of thirty days of not eating mush. Give yourself a couple of week, so that your body can adjust to the change.

After your thirty days you can in moderation begin three-meals a day in small portion with the list below. Keep in mind that your shed weight loss is beginning not over, you must continue it for five more months in moderation and eat sensible and in small portions. As stated before your body needs time to adjust to change of adding more food your meals. It's not the time to indulge you are still determine to shed some weight, so pray and continue to seek God for strength and guidance.

It is good to wait another week, before you eat a complete meal, you don't want to jump right into this, give your mind and body a space to accommodate the change.

This is the food items for the five-month ahead shed weight loss journey after the thirty days

Meats, mall portion of chicken, fish, steak, tuna, and ground chuck.
Beans
Rice

Green peas or beans (optional)
Vegetables (small portion)
Fruits (one or two) a day
Cottage cheese/ with any fruits and raisins
Small amount of grits and butter/with 1 sausage (your choice)
Small portion of toast wheat bread twice a week (optional)
Small amount of sweet only once a week (optional)
Snapple drinks
Water (8 glasses) a day
Cinnamon tea

Although you are now ready to add others or more foods to your menu, you much remember that you need to be sensible and eat in moderation, because you cannot go the extra mile due to what you starting out to do.

Your goal is to lose weight and you must stay focus and learn to eat small portion of the above menu for the five-months that is ahead. I will give you an example of what I did for the five months. That first month I only ate some of the thirty-day menu and included some off the items in the five-month menu each week. For instance, the second month I included for breakfast: coffee with honey, cream and grits with eggs and cheese.

I never had a desire for cakes, cookies, ice cream, candies and cold drinks, because I know that these will cause you to over indulge and most of all gain weight. So you need to keep a record of all that you eat in you thirty-day menu and the five-month menu. The weight will shed, believe me I am a living witness it work. You may or may not know that I have a television program and television make you look larger than you are, but the thirty-days really cause me to be so happy in mind and body when I had the chance to see me on television and the weight was gone.

Just remember this is not a diet, pray and seek God face for His help to get you from what used to have you bound and enslave, so that you can reach your promise land of health and slim.

Food you can eat after the three month, only in moderation, remember you have come this far, the food is now available, but eat sensible if you are determine to keep the weight off. Remember cold drinks whether diet or not they cause you to gain, so please avoid it if all possible. None of these food, is diet, so please be careful of what you eat, all foods listed in this book is natural foods not diets food.

Meats, only once a week if need be
Sweets, any kind (optional) very small portion
Cold drinks (optional) I prefer you to Snapple
Breads, any kind (optional) one slice
Candies (stay away from if possible)
Potatoes (optional) very fatness
Fried food (once a week if need be)
Potato chips (optional) only five if need be
Ice cream (optional) if need be

There are no diet foods to buy, just eat the food listed in this book and your pocketbook will not suffer. Most of the food listed in the book you buy for your grocery list. When you feel as if you are going to indulge please remember to seek the face of God. You must persist from the first day you started this pounds loss for the journey to lose the weight you so desired.

CHAPTER 9

"What to do, when you don't know, what to do"

YOU KNOW IT'S amazing when you are involve in doing something that you enjoy, such as walking or runner or just setting and thinking, and a solution come to mind of something you have been really trying to figure out, like losing weight and you began to picture it as your life answer to the problem. That's really intrigue me and I began to pen this solution, I believe what we do when we are dedicated to doing a thing that is benefited to our lives as a whole we try to work it out, even when we don't know what to do. I picture a waterfall where the water was flickering, sparkling, blue, beautiful, and there I was looking to see if I could visualize the answer to the problem of what to do, for instant you want to lose weight. As I continue to wonder and began to utilize every thought that came to my mind, I remember a beautiful story in the Bible in 2 Chronicle 20 chapter, where Jehoshaphat was told that a great multitude was coming against him. And he feared, but he seeks the face of God for an answer, fear began to grip his heart, he at the moment did not know what to do.

As sometime in our lives we are face with many things, which baffle us to the point of not knowing what to do, let's look at the weight problems we face today in our society, and in our personal lives. We have struggle, became frustrated and said things as "what the used, or I give up, because we really did not know what to do. Well I got the answer in this book to help solve the problems. You know as Jehoshaphat and his people prayed to God, there came an answer, God spoke to Jahaziel and said, be not afraid nor dismayed by reason of this great multitude, for the battle is not yours, but God. You see we can't just lose weight by looking at it, or by not eating (very danger to our health).

God had a plan for his people just like He used Jahaziel to help the Israelites. He are the same caring God today. When someone cried out to God for a need, He always has a solution, remember there is never a problem with God, He always have a solution. That solution and plan was in the heart of someone who dares to step forth and believe God for the answer in the all-natural healthy way to lose weight. She steps out on prayer as Jehoshaphat did and God by His power (Holy Spirit) gave her the unction of the Holy Spirit to spread the new in a simple and natural menu that we all can afford. God told Jehoshaphat to stand still and see the salvation of His Power, He gave them the strength to win the battle, so stand firm and see how God will bring you through to your weight loss desire. So as you read this book and apply it to your situation of losing weights, stand on God Word to see you through to your desire goal. So what do you do, when you do know what to do, just pray and believe God and His strength to guide you through to your promise land?

Menus

Breakfast	Lunch	Dinner
Grits with butter	Tuna salad	
Eggs	Crackers	Ground beef
Sausages	Snapple drink	Peas
Orange juice	Water	Corn
Water		Snapple drink
	Green salad	
Cottage cheese	Cracker	Fried tomatoes
Any Fruits	Water	Cracker
Water		Water
	Bake chicken	
Oatmeal	Rice	Baked turkey
Orange juice	Peas	Cabbage
Water	Water	Sweet potatoes (small portion)
Cereals (optional)	Fish	Water
Fruits	Baked beans	
Water	Corns	Steak
	Snapple drink	Rice
		Greens
Yoplait yogurt		
Water		

BENEFIT OF CINNAMON TEA

CINNAMON: CINNAMON WAS one of the first trade spices of the ancient world. Biblical references indicate that merchants carried the Asian spice all the way from Ceylon to Palestine. The English word cinnamon derives from the Hebrew word Cinnamon, and the spice is mentioned in Psalms, Proverbs, Ezekiel, and Revelations. Moses, the patriarch of patriarchs, commanded the children of Israel to anoint the tabernacle, the vessels of the tabernacle, and the priests themselves with ointments made of cinnamon.

Cinnamon is one of the oldest tonic plants on the globe. The world may not agree politically, but in the realm of tonics, all acknowledge that cinnamon is good for health. The daily use of cinnamon could well improve your health, it really has improved mine, and I have been drinking cinnamon tea since 1997. The Chinese believe that cinnamon heats up a cold body, improves the circulation, and generally gets the blood rushing around, stoking up the waning fire, if you will, and they prescribe it for loss of vigor, whether due to stress, aging, or illness. They believe the tea warms the kidneys and cures impotence, weak legs, and backache. Specifically, cinnamon is held supreme for blood deficiencies that leave one feeling weak.

My experience of using cinnamon tea is that it really helps the body to rejuvenated, help backaches; help strengthen weak legs, fever, and upset stomach. Cinnamon gets rid of the bad things that hang out in the stomach, calms it down, and makes it stronger.

Notes

Notes

Notes

Notes

www.ingramcontent.com/pod-product-compliance
Lightning Source LLC
Chambersburg PA
CBHW050341290526
45785CB00006B/2582